Christopher A. Pickard

Hack Your Way to Lower Blood Pressure

7 Effective Lifestyle Strategies To Treat Hypertension

First edition

This book was professionally typeset on Reedsy
Find out more at reedsy.com

'Self-peace starts with self-health'
- Chris Pickard, 2018

"If there is righteousness in the heart, there will be beauty in the character.
If there is beauty in the character, there will be harmony in the home.
If there is harmony in the home, there will be order in the nations.
When there is order in the nations, there will peace in the world."

— Confucius

Contents

Foreword....................1
Preface....................3
Introduction....................4
I. PART ONE....................7
1. My Father's Story....................8
2. Why should you worry about high blood pressure, and what causes it?....................12
3. Happy Beautiful Day....................18
4. 'Normal' does not equal 'Healthy'....................24
5. It's Genetic – No it's probably not!....................27
6. The big problem with drugs – and why being on them 'forever' without a VERY good reason may be a mistake....................30
II. PART 2: THE MAGNIFICENT 7 HEALTH STRATEGIES FOR OPTIMAL BLOOD PRESSURE....................35
7. This is not everything.......................36
8. Hydration....................38
9. Nitric Oxide: 'Talk Right'....................40
10. Modified Mediterranean 'Paleo NO' DASH Diet: Eat Right....................49
11. Detox 'the 10 Day Blood Pressure Blitz'....................56
12. Resilience to Stress: Think Right....................59
13. Circadian Rhythm: Better Sleep....................63
14. The Goldilocks Exercise Program....................68
15. Health Span vs Life Span....................71
III. THE ASSESSMENT & RESOURCES....................74
16. The Magnificent 7 Lifestyle Screening Assessment....................75
17. What's Next?....................81
18. About the Author....................83
1.
2.
3.

4.

5.

6.

7.

8.

9.

10.

11.

12.

13.

14.

15.

16.

17.

18.

19.

20.

21.

22.

23.

Foreword

'Happy Beautiful Day' is a phrase I picked up from one of the world's greatest doctors....

On the 22nd April 2014 I thought I knew a lot about health and well being.

I had traveled the world and spent thousands and thousands of pounds educating myself about all aspects of health.

I'd learned from many different people, including chiropractors, osteopaths, nutritionists, spiritual healers, yogi's, herbalists, medical doctors, neurologists, and even a very fine cardiologist.

I had helped people improve their health and get off pain killers, blood pressure medication, cholesterol medication and blood sugar medication.

Surely I knew something?

On the morning of the 23rd of April, at a business breakfast meeting of all things, I met Pete Cohen, one of the world's top life coaches, who was soon going to introduce me to how little I knew.

Pete and I hit it off straight away (down to his amazing communication skills and infectious enthusiasm) and became friends pretty much instantly, which is why 1 month later, on a beautiful sunny Friday lunchtime I was sitting in Pete's garden discussing nutrition with an extraordinary man from Huston, Texas: Dr Bob Rakowski.

Dr Bob Rakowski spent many years teaching medical doctors and other health practitioners, with the founder of Functional Medicine - Dr Jeff Bland. Dr Bland had been the head of research for the Linus Pauling institute (Linus Pauling had won 2 Noble Prizes!)

'Dr Bob' had played a crucial role in helping Pete's fiancé (now wife) Hannah, regain her health after experimental cancer treatment for terminal brain cancer. Dr Bob had taught Hannah a series of strategies that transformed her body from being a 'host for disease' to a 'host for life'.

Having one such story is great, but Dr Bob has helped hundreds, if not thousands overcome and reverse seemingly impossible health challenges. This impressive track record got me hooked on learning all I could about these strategies so I could help my own patients more profoundly.

There are seven strategies, which Dr Bob refers to as 'The Magnificent 7', and you'll learn about them in this book, and how to apply them to optimizing blood pressure.

Preface

How To Use This Book

I really want you to be able to take swift action on the aspects of your lifestyle that may be conspiring with any genetic or familial issues you have (see later for the true science on genetics), so I've created a short, mildly scientifically verified, assessment for you to take.

So my quick advice is to skip to the 'Magnificent 7 Lifestyle Assessment' at the end of the book, figure out which areas need the most work, then read the specific segments of Part 2 of the book to take action.

Then come back and carry on reading the rest.

The very fact that you are reading this book tells me you probably don't need to know 'why' you need to treat blood pressure naturally, so the first section of this book is for information purposes only.

So please take the assessment, take action, and you can reach out to me personally if you wish to share your success, or get stuck or find major errors or problems: beatbloodpressure@gmail.com

Serving Your Wellness,

Chris Pickard

Introduction

If you suspect your blood pressure today is the result of the decisions you've made in the past, you are almost certainly correct. It's likely that you don't know for sure what those decisions where though, which is why you are reading this.

The good news is you are about to find out, so you can start making better decisions today that lower your blood pressure tomorrow. (OK, maybe not exactly tomorrow, but if you consistently apply better habits, you will get the reward)

Modern medicine ensures you are likely going to live 80 or 90 years, and possibly 100.

Unfortunately, this increase in longevity is not brought about by making us more robust and healthier, but my allowing us to 'limp along further' in an ever more decayed state.

This is because medicine focuses on disease. Everyone gets treated the same, and you can only get treated if you have something wrong.

Even vaccines don't actually build health – they merely try to prevent one disease at a time.

There is however another way.

All the major chronic diseases such as cancer, heart disease, diabetes, lung disease, dementia, Alzheimer's, Parkinson's and High Blood Pressure are only partially genetic.

Up to 90% are caused by your choices and your environment. If you take control of your choices and teach your family and friends about what you learn, you will avert the causes of death of 90% of the population and become one of the privileged that lives to a 'ripe' old age with vigour, vitality and clarity and add an extra 20 years to your 'health span'.

Who Am I?

I'm a Doctor of Chiropractic. A member the International Association of Functional Neurology, I'm the first and maybe only UK trained member of the Cardiovascular Health Institute, and I wake up every morning to inspire everyone to better health to the future, and I also very passionate about the world peace process ...

I believe that world peace starts with self-peace, and self-peace starts with self-health. And if we all look after ourselves in a deeper, more meaningful way, it's going to have a greater effect on our own self peace and our self-worth, and that's going to help us spread self-peace and self-worth to other people. Maybe, maybe we're going to actually change the minds of some of the people making crazy decisions at the moment in the world.

I also have my picture in the Guinness Book of Records, the 2014 addition, page 70. It's very small, but I am in there.

DISCLAIMER

This book is more informational purposes only and expresses the opinion of the author based on scientific findings and also mentoring from cardiologists and functional medical doctors.

The book itself is not to diagnose prevent or cure any disease. Please speak with your healthcare provider regarding any change in your health and wellness care plan.

I

Part One

"The problem with our health care system is that you have to lose your health to enter it."
Dr Dean Black

The Myths and the Problems With Conventional Hypertension Treatment.

And an Introduction to The Magnificent 7.

1

My Father's Story

Almost 50% of the US adult population have hypertension (it's similar in the UK where I am). About a quarter have arthritis. A fifth have respiratory diseases. Chronic mental conditions, and general heart disease combined is 10-15%.

So, half of all adults have some level of high blood pressure, and it's linked to some major problems (even when 'controlled' by drugs).

<u>My Father's Story</u>

So why am I so interested in heart disease and high blood pressure? Well, all my grandparents suffered to some degree with these, and then there's my father.

Now, my father when he was in his 50's (which is what I am now), had never been overweight, he's not been completely sedentary, he has always loved walking, but he started getting high blood pressure and then high blood sugar, partly possibly because of side effects to the high blood drugs, but that's another story.

It's the same story actually, which we will get to in a moment.

When he came in to my clinic to have his neck manipulated his blood pressure would go down. (It turns out that a lot of people have high blood pressure because of neck pain and neck problems. It is documented that massage therapy on the neck can actually help, and there are some trials that show that appropriate chiropractic care can actually help lower blood pressure in some people).

As a brief aside, I actually have a patient at the moment, that when we look after his neck, his blood sugar has also decreased, which brings me back to my father and his blood sugar.

Now, my father's high blood pressure was only temporarily helped by chiropractic, and as time went on his blood sugar also went up (and up). Despite the medication, and despite the advice he was following from the dietitians on the NHS, his blood sugar was getting higher and higher. It was so bad that the pills weren't keeping that under control and my father was told he would need insulin in a month's time. Insulin is the drug that your pancreas makes to control blood sugar by getting it into your cells and out of your blood.

My Dad was not at all happy with this, so he asked, "What else can we do?" And luckily, I'd just attended a seminar with Dr James Chesnut, and I said, "Here Dad, why don't we try this?". So he followed a very strict diet - he basically only ate raw vegetables and some raw fruit, with occasional eggs and meat, but not very much. Also no alcohol, no tea, no coffee (I allowed him to have one cup of tea per day) and I was very, very strict. And after two weeks, my Dad's blood pressure and blood sugar actually came down to good numbers, but still on the drugs.

My Dad being my Dad, he didn't' like taking drugs, and so without consulting his doctor, weaned himself off of the drugs over the next week to see what would happen, and after three weeks he had completely normal blood pressure and normal blood sugar without any drugs. And then after four weeks, it was all still completely normal, and he went back to his doctor.

Do Doctors Want To Know The Truth?

After seeing my father's new readings, the doctor said, "Ah, fantastic Mr. Pickard, the medication is finally working." Then my dad said, "Actually, no. I stopped the medication one week ago, and everything's been fine for the past two weeks because of the diet that my son put me on".

At this point, someone truly interested in the health and wellbeing of their patients would ask 'what was the diet?', but as I have come to discover, many of today's busy, overworked doctors don't have time to learn about, and then educate their patients. So, my father's doctor, didn't ask a single question about what he had done, he may as well of put a paper bag over his head and stuck his fingers in his ears, he just went, "Oh," and that was it.

He didn't want to know what my father had done, didn't ask any details at all, didn't want to pass it on to any patients, seemed to be completely uninterested in the fact that this was a 'miracle', as far as he was concerned.

And this, I've come to learn over the past 20 years, is pretty much, how many doctors, and also many patients, are actually responding. They don't want to know that they don't have to take drugs, and that their disease is not necessarily a disease, it's a lifestyle problem.

What I'm hoping is that you ARE interested in making some changes, and my sincere wish is that by reading this book, you will have the knowledge that you need to achieve great levels of health, no matter where you are now, and actually add 20 years of health to your life.

2

Why should you worry about high blood pressure, and what causes it?

7% of the US adult population have heart disease, and it is the number one killer in the world. It's on the rise, and what's leading the chart as a cause of heart disease is high blood pressure.

Blood pressure is the leading cause of strokes and heart disease, and more and more people have high blood pressure all the time, every year, despite supposedly healthy low-fat diets, and more and more medication.

High blood pressure is linked to damage and degeneration in every organ of the body, like the brain, eyes and kidneys.

While it's commonly known that which blood pressure can cause these problems, what is not commonly known, and often missed, is that the underlying cause of the high blood pressure can also be causing these problems.

So while a drug may lower blood pressure, it may not be treating the actual cause of the damage, so the damage keeps occurring.

Also, blood pressure is happening younger, and younger, and younger, and it's not because our genetics are changing...

... so it is becoming more and more apparent that the current ways medicine is treating blood pressure is not really helping.

Time to meet the doctor of the future.

"The doctor of the future will give no medication but will interest his patients in the care of the human frame, diet and in the cause and prevention of disease"—Thomas A. Edison

Now, Mr. Edison was not a doctor. But he was a very, very clever man, and he predicted that if you do the right things, you don't need medicine. Unfortunately, doctors are not taught how to help patients not need medicine!

It's hardly surprising though because it's easier to pop a pill than it is to change your habits, and even if doctors did learn about how to achieve optimal health, it's human nature to take the easy path.

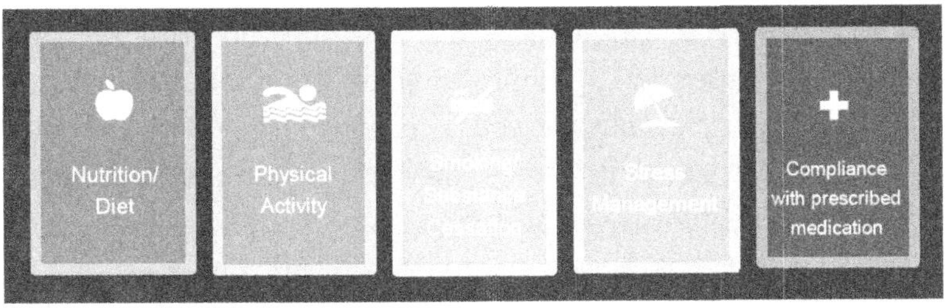

Now, if you do go to the doctor with blood pressure, there are five major areas that doctors should be looking at right away.

The first point is nutrition and diet. Your eating pattern is the number one way that you can change your blood pressure. A healthy eating plan is actually more powerful than medicine, more than is commonly recognized. It's often the place to start with many of today's chronic health issues. It could be something you are eating, something you are NOT eating, or even how or when you eat (where to start is coming later in the book).

Unfortunately it's more than likely that your doctor, apart from saying, 'just eat healthy, and eat less salt', doesn't have any advice about what you should be eating. While too much salt can be a cause of high blood pressure, it is by no means the only cause.

Medical doctors are generally not the best people to ask about healthy diet, as they learn about disease, medicine and surgery, not health. In fact, if you look at their diet, it's probably similar to yours. They mayeven be on blood pressure medication themselves because they didn't realise what they thought of as a healthy balanced diet, was anything but healthy and balanced.

No.2 is physical activity...

Physical Activity, again, it's very unlikely that the doctor will actually give you any real advice on how to promote your physical activities or to improve your strength, and what is worse, they may encourage you to exercise beyond your body's capacity to repair which may then cause even higher blood pressure. Which is why I encourage 'the Goldilocks' approach to exercise, which is about getting it just right for you.

I want to make it clear here that I am in no way trying to put down conventional medicine. Medical doctors are the best people in the world for saving your life if you are in serious trouble! They have the best training.

The problem is medical training does not incorporate health building, lifestyle, nutrition, exercise and the impact of environmental toxins on our health (and what to do about it).

Treating disease with drugs and surgery is a very different job from building health and longevity.

Next – 'stop smoking, and drink less alcohol' (and maybe less caffeine). I'm sure nobody in this day and age needs to go to a medical practitioner to know smoking and drinking are harmful. But did you know that caffeine is only a problem for some? And that in most people coffee and tea can actually be protective in the long run? Alcohol and smoking are two well know toxins, but there are many, many more in our environment that are causing high blood pressure by stealth. The air you breath, the chemicals you clean with, and even medication you are taking for something else, are all toxins that can, and do, cause high blood pressure in millions of people. The home you live in can even be 'growing' the cause of your hypertension.

All these causes you have not been checked for may be causing you a little stress about now, which brings me to factor number 4 – stress.

While stress is recognised as a major contributing cause of high blood pressure, it's often unlikely that you'll be referred for any kind of stress management courses, counseling, or introduced to positive psychology tools.

Now we get to the final option, which is really the only course of action that doctors have training in with blood pressure, and that's compliance with prescribed medication.

And because doctors have very little training on the first 4, and they really want to help you, they go all in on what they know best, which is often not what you, the patient wants to know.

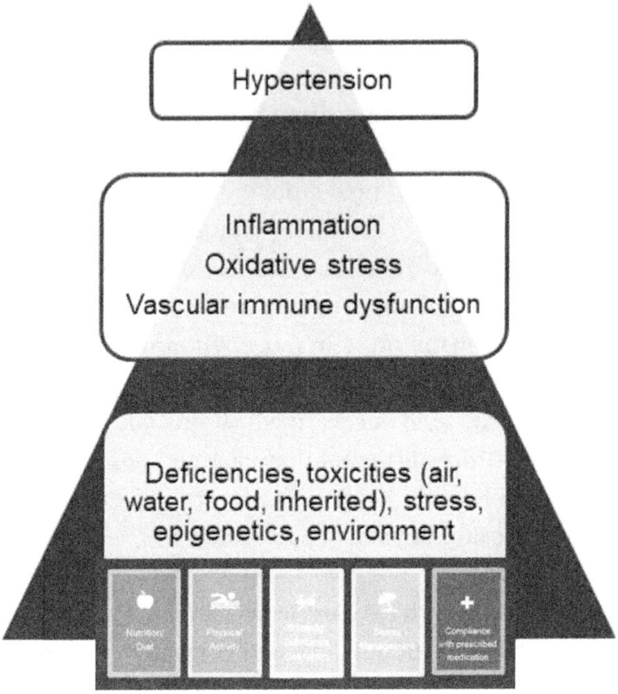

Let's dive a little deeper.

High blood pressure itself is, according to a new emerging model for integrated medical doctors in the United States, caused by three major things:

- inflammation in the body (think of it like fire in the body)
- oxidative stress in the body (imagine a process like rusting)
- and vascular immune dysfunction

We're going to come back to that last one in a moment.

These 3 things, inflammation, oxidative stress, and vascular immune dysfunction, are themselves caused by other things, such as poor nutrition or deficiencies; toxicities including air pollution, water pollution, food pollution, and toxicities you inherit from your mother, and even your grandmother (toxins like lead get passed from mother to child); stress; epigenetics (which is how your genes actually change with what you do); and then the environment itself.

It's because high blood pressure has so many causes, that it's easier just to treat the end result.

But this is actually dangerous, as blood pressure pills don't treat any of the underlying causes, so the inflammation, oxidation and vascular dysfunction spreads, and causes other problems – such as kidney or liver disease, dementia, or cancers.

So what can be done differently?

Well, what I do with my patients is introduce them to something called the magnificent seven health strategies that I learned from one of my mentors...

3

Happy Beautiful Day

'Happy Beautiful Day' is a phrase I picked up from one of the world's greatest doctors....

On the 22nd April 2014 I thought I knew a lot about health and wellbeing.

I had traveled the world and spent thousands and thousands of pounds on educating myself about all aspects of health. From chiropractors, osteopaths, nutritionists, spiritual healers, yogi's, herbalists, medical doctors, neurologists, and even a very fine cardiologist. I had helped many, including my father, avoid insulin and even get off blood pressure medication.

Surely I knew something?

On the morning of the 23rd of April, at a business breakfast meeting of all things, I met Pete Cohen, one of the world's top life coaches, who was soon going to introduce me to how little I knew.

Pete and I hit it off straight away (down to his amazing communication skills and infectious enthusiasm) and became friends pretty much instantly, which is why 1 month later, on a beautiful sunny Friday lunchtime I was sitting in Pete's garden discussing nutrition with an extraordinary man from Huston, Texas: Dr Bob Rakowski.

Dr Bob Rakowski spent many years teaching medical doctors and other health practitioners, with the founder of Functional Medicine - Dr Jeff Bland. Dr Bland had been the head of research for the Linus Pauling institute (Linus Pauling had won 2 Noble Prizes!)

'Dr Bob' had played a crucial role in helping Pete's fiancé (now wife) Hannah, regain her health after experimental cancer treatment for terminal brain cancer. Dr Bob had taught Hannah a series of strategies that transformed her body from being a 'host for disease' to a 'host for life'.

Having one such story is great, but Dr Bob has helped hundreds, if not thousands overcome and reverse seemingly impossible health challenges. This impressive track record got me hooked on learning all I could about these strategies so I could help my own patients more profoundly.

There are seven strategies, which Dr Bob refers to as 'The Magnificent 7'.

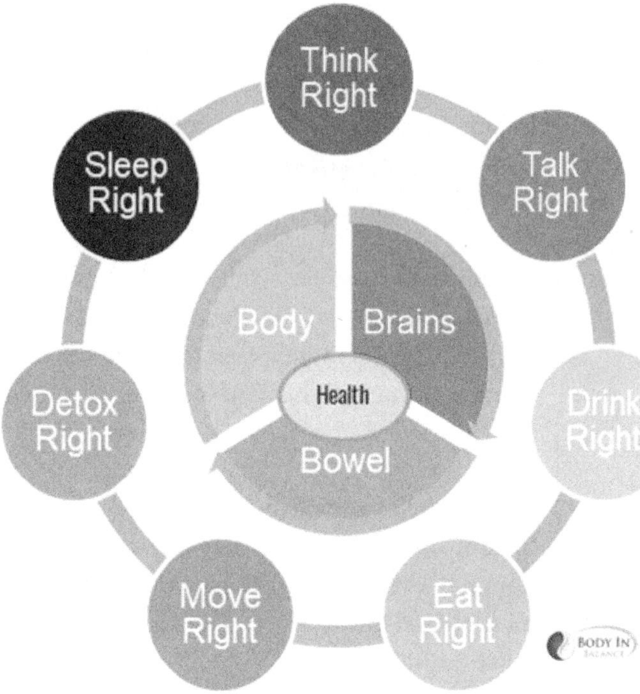

Dr Rakowski, aka Dr Bob, was inspired in part by Steven Covey's book, "The 7 Habits of Highly Effective People", and the classic cowboy film The Magnificent 7, which itself was inspired by an older Japanese film The 7 Samurai.

Dr Rakowski works with everyone from people who have been told to 'go home and die' as they have no hope of rescue from conventional medicine, to US Olympic and Sports stars wanting to get more from their bodies. The Magnificent 7 works for them all, and they will work for you too.

1) Think Right

This is about making the right choices, as Dr Bob puts it 'Choose Health. Choose Life!' Take the time to reflect on any decisions you make, are they life affirming, or health sapping? This applies to food choices, exercise, relationships, even business and work. Every decision you make leads you down a path. It's your responsibility to learn how to choose wisely, and healthily. The good news about 'bad' decisions is you can learn from them and change your mind.

I really love this quote from Brendon Burchard, "When your mind gets right, your life gets right."

Focus on becoming a 'Wonderful, warm human being'

And here is a Hebrew word (I think) that I really liked the meaning of, that helps remind me to think like a wonderful, warm, human being:

Tikkun - 'the mending of the world through intense soul-work and acts of creative love and justice'

2) Talk Right

Talking right is all about communication. Good communication leads to good relationships. This principle applies to communicating with other people, with your inner 'self-talk' and even deeper with all of your body's signaling systems. How your very cells 'talk' to each other effects your health – when it goes wrong this can lead to cancer and autoimmune disease for instance.

Dr Bob's top tip – laugh more. Laughter brings happiness to those that hear it, and it boosts your immune system to.

3) Eat Right

How far off the launch pad would a space rocket get if you didn't give it the right fuel? How long would a house last if you used poor building materials? Not very far/long in either case. The same is true of your body and mind. If you don't feed it what it really needs, then things will inevitably break down, or fail to repair at all. In this day and age, if you eat any less than 9 servings of fresh, organic veg and fruit, and you don't take supplements (there is a Magnificent 7 supplement list), you are likely to suffer some form of deficiency leading to more frequent acute and chronic illness.

Eating right, we have only recently rediscovered, is not only about what you eat, it's also about how and when you eat, each day and through the seasons. Getting the timing right is possibly the most powerful tool we have to both overcoming illness and maintaining optimal health.

4) Drink Right

As far as I'm aware, every chemical reaction in your body takes place in solution. As you'll find in out later, it doesn't have to be pure water to hydrate you, but certainly don't expect sugary, syrupy, energy drinks, or artificial flavours and sweeteners, to aid your chemical processes. My rule of thumb is if you have a glass of filtered water every hour or so and you pee it out within 30 minutes you are likely hydrated. If you exercise, or are talking lots or a mouth breather, then you will need to drink more water.

5) Move Right

Exercise is the best medicine. You've heard that before, I'm sure. Regular exercise boosts the immune system, turns off stress and makes you feel good. It literally nourishes every cell in your body and keeps you young. Move every joint and muscle every day in all directions to keep your machine well-oiled and ready for action!

6) Sleep Right

Dr Bob points out, you are either running on stress and adrenaline or rest and recovery. Without adequate sleep you cannot repair. A supportive mattress, the right pillow, your sleeping position, what time you go to bed, and what you do before going to bed all make a difference. Neglect healthy sleeping habits at your peril.

7) 'Poop' Right.

There's nothing to get embarrassed about here. We all do it.

When we talk 'poop' we mean everything involved in the elimination of toxins and waste from your body. So your gut, liver, kidneys, lungs and skin all need to be working optimally. Every single cell in your body creates waste and can be damaged by toxins, this is where your DNA is, so you must look after your cells to get well and stay well.

The Magnificent 7 Heroes protect your body, your brain and your bowels from stress, toxins and recover faster from trauma.

So now you know about the Magnificent 7 in general, what about a specialist 'mag 7' for lowering High Blood Pressure?

Before we get to that though, you may be thinking:

- The doctor tested everything and it all came back normal
- My problem is genetic
- Once you are on drugs you have to stay on them forever

So let's answer some of those before we continue...

4

'Normal' does not equal 'Healthy'

'Normal is not normal if you are not feeling normal' Dr McCullough

Has Your Doctor Told You Your Blood Test Came Back Normal?

I would hazard a guess that you have had at least one blood test from your doctor, and they said that it's all normal, nothings wrong, except maybe high cholesterol. You are put on a drug, but you don't feel better, and there's no explanation.

I've included a picture below of a normal blood test result from a real patient, in the UK. The 'normal' ranges listed on the right, that doctors use, are unfortunately based on outdated science. Worse, is that these ranges are in some cases, not just unhealthy, but dangerous.

'Normal' is not the same as Healthy

21-Oct-2020	Serum lipids - (AB8886) - Normal - No Action			
	HDL <1 mmol/L is a risk factor for coronary heart disease.			
	Serum cholesterol	4.7	mmol/L	
	Serum HDL cholesterol level	2.1	mmol/L	
	Serum cholesterol/HDL ratio	2.2		
21-Oct-2020	Liver function test - (AB8886) - Normal - No Action			
	AST serum level	14	u/L	<40.00u/L
	Serum ALT level	12	iu/L	<41.00iu/L
	Serum LDH level	283	u/L	240.00 - 480.00u/L
	Serum gamma GT level	15	u/L	1.00 - 60.00u/L
	Serum total bilirubin level	3	umol/L	<21.00umol/L
	Mean corpuscular volume (MCV)	94.9	fL	83.00 - 101.00fL
	Mean corpusc. haemoglobin(MCH)	31.5	pg	27.00 - 32.00pg
	Red blood cell distribut width	13.2	%	11.60 - 14.00%
	Platelet count	326	10*9/L	150.00 - 410.0010*9/L
	Neutrophil count	3.8	10*9/L	2.00 - 7.0010*9/L
	Lymphocyte count	1.1	10*9/L	1.00 - 3.0010*9/L
	Monocyte count	0.6	10*9/L	0.20 - 1.0010*9/L

What we now know, from extensive research in medical journals, is that the truly healthy levels are much narrower than the accepted 'normal' and it's often its not even in the middle of the normal range.

For instance, while the test results below were considered normal, and therefore 'nothing wrong', an updated analysis revealed quite a lot wrong (everything with a red arrow is potentially a warning sign related to increased disease incidence.

The red lines indicate 'out of healthy'

21-Oct-2020		Serum lipids - (AB8886) - Normal - No Action			
		HDL <1 mmol/L is a risk factor for coronary heart disease.			
		Serum cholesterol	4.7	mmol/L	
	→	Serum HDL cholesterol level	2.1	mmol/L	
		Serum cholesterol/HDL ratio	2.2		
21-Oct-2020		Liver function test - (AB8886) - Normal - No Action			
		AST serum level	14	u/L	<40.00u/L
		Serum ALT level	12	iu/L	<41.00iu/L
	→	Serum LDH level	283	u/L	240.00 - 480.00u/L
		Serum gamma GT level	15	u/L	1.00 - 60.00u/L
	→	Serum total bilirubin level	3	umol/L	<21.00umol/L
	→	Mean corpuscular volume (MCV)	94.9	fL	83.00 - 101.00fL
		Mean corpusc. haemoglobin(MCH)	31.5	pg	27.00 - 32.00pg
	→	Red blood cell distribut width	13.2	%	11.60 - 14.00%
	→	Platelet count	326	10*9/L	150.00 - 410.0010*9/L
	→	Neutrophil count	3.8	10*9/L	2.00 - 7.0010*9/L
		Lymphocyte count	1.1	10*9/L	1.00 - 3.0010*9/L
	→	Monocyte count	0.6	10*9/L	0.20 - 1.0010*9/L

So the doctor tells the patient 'there is nothing wrong', and then the patient goes away frustrated because they can feel in themselves that something is wrong. The reality is though, that in just about every blood test I've seen on a patient, there really IS something wrong, and then there is direct action to take.

Of course, it is entirely possible that the patient could feel fine, the only issue being high blood pressure. And the blood test above actually revealed some of the potential areas that if fixed, would improve blood pressure (and they actually did)

However, you can't rely on only a few markers in the blood test, it does get a bit more complicated...

You see some things that are bad for us, and some diseases, lower some of our blood test numbers; and there are some things that can raise these numbers. So you can actually have two things that are bad for you/wrong with you; one that's lowering the numbers and one that's raising the numbers, and so your blood results can look completely normal and healthy.

Luckily if your doctor does the right history and asks the right questions, you can uncover what's going on, get further tests if needed; and then you can actually fix what's really going on.

The big lesson here, is to find out how long your doctor takes to analyse your test results, and if it's only a cursory glance, get a second opinion.

As far as I'm concerned the best blood chemistry analysis training is delivered by Dr Bryan Walsh of Metabolic Fitness in the USA. try and find someone trained by him. (I'm biased because he was one of people I learned from).

5

It's Genetic – No it's probably not!

Let's talk about genetics.

I know a lot of people really think that their health problem is genetic, because their parents had it and their grandparents had it, so it seems logical.

However, there is a big difference between what people think of as genetic, and what is really going on here, which is 'epigenetic'.

In basic terms it means that your family has a predisposition to develop a disease IF they don't get enough of the right nutrients, or lead the right lifestyle.

So, if you lead the right lifestyle, and have all the right nutrients you will not flip on the epigenetic switch.

The PREDICT Study

Professor Tim Spector runs the biggest twin study in the world and a couple of my patients are actually in that study.

It consists of 13,000 twins, many of them are identical.

Now, the thing about identical twins is they have identical genetics, so that means there's no genetic difference between them. Yet they found that one twin could have all kinds of health problems, heart disease and high blood pressure for instance, while the other one can be completely fine.

What they discovered was that the health of the individual is more down to what they eat and how that changes their the gut bacteria, the microbiome.

So the current conclusion of the Twin study is that what you do, and what you eat, is more a predictor of your health and disease state than your genetics. So even if everyone else in your family has high blood pressure, and your doctor says 'it's genetic' there is almost certainly something positive you can do.

Eating and lifestyle trumps genetics.

Dr Dean Ornish

Dean Ornish is another scientist looking at genetics versus lifestyle. His big study focused on prostate health. Dr Ornish put men through a 90-day health, wellness and lifestyle program. And after 90 days, about 400 genes were changed, more healthy genes got switched on, some of the unhealthy ones got switched off. And this is due to through diet and the lifestyle. 90 days completely changed how people's DNA was being expressed.

8 Weeks To A Younger You

This is a more recent study and I was really exciting because the products that were used where close to those I recommend to patients.

This study put a group of people through an eight-week program, including diet, sleep, exercise, and relaxation guidelines, as well as supplemental probiotics and phytonutrients (coloured nutrients you find in plants).

Before the study they measured everyone's 'genetic age', and then measured again 8 weeks later.

On average everyone became genetically younger by 3.2 years.

So, altering lifestyle factor in multiple areas can make you three years younger in just eight weeks.

Imagine if you followed this program for a year, how much better you would feel.

Sounds like a great treatment option to me.

6

The big problem with drugs – and why being on them 'forever' without a VERY good reason may be a mistake

The big problem is that the drugs don't work, not in the way you want them to.

Blood pressure drugs are actually failing quite miserably to tackle the underlying problem.

The amount of people with high blood pressure is rising and heart disease is still going up, despite more drugs. With those on medication, only 34% of people respond favourably, i.e. a single drug brings the blood pressure under control.

34% seems much better than nothing, but seeing as 'placebo' (a pill with no active ingredient) works 33% of the time, it's not that much better than nothing.

What's more, according to one survey, 97% of people report significant side effects to medication. 50%-80% of patients are not compliant with treatment and 40% discontinue treatment due to the side effects.

Many people, doctors included, think that if they stop taking their blood pressure pills, that they're going to have a heart attack or stroke and die in the next few days, and you've got to take them every single day because the drugs lower the blood pressure, and that's what actually helps you.

The truth of the matter however is somewhat different.

According to research available at www.nnt.com, over a 5 year period, only 1 in 67 people will have a stroke prevented, 1 in 100 will have a heart attack prevented and 1 in 125 will have their life saved by taking blood pressure drugs.

Now if you are that 1 person, then great, and certainly to have SOME chance of prevention is better than nothing, but believing drugs are the best answer is simply not true.

There are still a lot of deaths, strokes, and heart attacks, in the people taking drugs. Looking at overall deaths, there was just slightly less deaths in the medicated group than the people not taking drugs.

So, on an individual basis, medication doesn't make a huge difference. But on a population level it makes enough of a difference for conventional medicine to carry on doing 'drugs first'.

The reason why drugs, by the themselves, don't really work for everyone is because medicine mostly focuses its effort and drugs on the RAAS system (the renin-angiotensin-aldosterone system).

Sodium – Not just a cause of High Blood Pressure

If you've watched as many wildlife documentaries as I have, then you'll know that animals deliberately seek out salt, and there are numerous 'salt licks' in the wild where animals congregate to get this vital mineral.

So why is salt so important?

Sodium is used in so many different ways in the body. It's used in every single cell.

Without sodium, you can't absorb vital nutrients from the food you eat.

So, if you have no sodium, your whole body stops working.

And it's so important that your body will do things to basically make sure you keep salt in your body.

For instance, where salt goes, water follows, and your blood needs a certain amount of salt (sodium) in it to draw in water. If you have low sodium, you'll have less water in your blood, and this will result in low blood pressure. With low blood pressure, you'll not be able to move vital nutrients to organs such as your brain.

So your kidneys have sensors that detect when the pressure is low, and then secrete a chemical called renin. The liver, if it's properly working, will convert that into angiotensinogen, which then converts to angiotensin 1. Then your lungs secrete something called ACE, the angiotensin-converting enzyme, to turn angiotensin I into angiotensin II. That then goes to your adrenal glands, (your 'get up and go' glands) and they make something called aldosterone, and aldosterone then tells your kidneys to increase sodium and water retention.

If you didn't follow that, don't worry, there are some great animations and videos on the internet you can search for.

The end result is you increase sodium and water retention, you basically get 'more stuff' in your blood, so your blood pressure can go up. And also, what happens is angiotensin tells your nervous system to constrict your blood vessels to make them smaller and tighter so there's less room for the fluids. So it all increases your blood pressure, so you can pump nutrients to your brain for instance.

So this whole system is in place to protect you from dehydration and low salt.

Because in nature, low blood pressure is far more of a threat to your life than high blood pressure.

But in today's society, people tend have too much salt. There is speculation that it may actually not be the sodium, it may be the chloride part of sodium chloride, which is common table salt (and it is quite unnatural). If you are going to use salt, make sure its rock salt or sea salt, not sodium chloride.

For now, let's stick to the current theory. If sodium goes too high, then your blood pressure is going to go too high, because too much water is drawn in to your arteries. Or if you haven't got enough of water, the blood becomes too thick, and it's harder to 'push'.

So the drugs that we have include renin inhibitors, ACE inhibitors, ARB inhibitors, and they stop this RAAS mechanism in various ways.

Even if you've got normal blood pressure and you take some of these drugs, your blood pressure will probably go down because you are inhibiting your normal mechanisms for keeping your blood pressure where it should be.

So even if you haven't got high salt, your blood pressure can go down if you take these drugs.

The problem is that for many people, their high blood pressure hasn't got anything to do with salt.

And so they can take a drug, it can lower their blood pressure, but the real reason that they've got high blood pressure is still there, so their blood pressure stays high, or goes high again soon. So they take another drug, which may lower their blood pressure or it may not, and they need another drug, and it just goes on and on and on and on.

...and every drug causes its own side effects, and can cause vital nutrient depletions, that then ironically leads to ... higher blood pressure.

So have a think. What kind of treatment advice would you like? Drugs that may give you a slightly decreased chance of dying, or a program that actually reverses the disease process itself? Or a combination of both, knowing that at some point you won't need the drugs?

Now we've covered two big myths, 'it's genetic so I can do nothing except take drugs' and 'drugs are the most important part of treatment', we can move on to fixing what is really wrong.

II

PART 2: The Magnificent 7 Health Strategies for Optimal Blood Pressure

"Everyone has imperfect chemistry ...
Performance improves as chemistry improves..."
Dr Bob Rakowski

7

This is not everything…

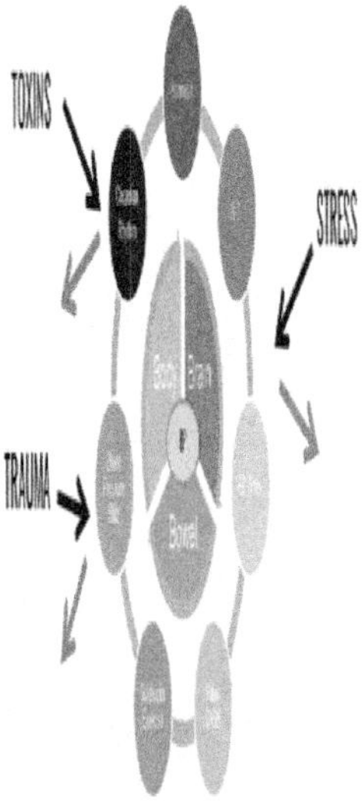

There are hundreds, if not thousands of vitamins, minerals, herbs, diets, relaxation techniques, physical therapies, and devices that can help optimise blood pressure.

Any one of them could give you a ‘cure’ or it may be that you need to do a number of things at once.

Taking a more strategic approach, such as that offered by 'The Mag 7' gives you your best shot of finding the right tracks swiftly.

What follows is not an exhaustive list of what can be done, and it may not be in the order of what I would suggest for you if we were working 1 to 1, but it's a sensible series of strategies.

Remember, if you are using this approach to lessen your need for medication PLEASE work with your doctor.

Now that is said, please start with the areas indicated by the Assessment.

8

Hydration

When the blood becomes thicker, it becomes harder to circulate, leading to higher blood pressure.

However, dehydration can also cause low blood pressure!

Top tip: unstable blood pressure may be a sign of dehydration.

True hydration is about far more than drinking water.

If you suspect hydration is your biggest issue then I may direct you to the best book on the subject, Quench.

Some of what the author reveals may surprise you.

Before I ever read Quench I was advising my patients to 'eat your water'.

Why?

Because fresh, uncooked vegetables and fruit are full of water that is usually of higher quality than what you find in your taps!

It's also because food sources of water contain something called 'exclusion zone water' or EZ water for short. EZ water is also known as structured water and living water.

EZ water exists as a gell, and helps line all your blood vessels and may actually help propel blood along your capillaries and take pressure off your heart.

EZ water may also be part of the mechanism that allows Nitric Oxide to help dilate your blood vessels and lower blood pressure (see later)

As well as eating whole plant foods, drinking water is still a good idea, but if you read Quench you'll also learn about the magic of adding chia seeds to water, why gentle movement is so important and so much more.

As simple hydration plan would be to include some raw food with every meal; try a tea spoon to a tablespoon of ground chia seeds in water 2 x day; and drink 2 or 3 big glasses of water with maybe a twist of lemon or lime juice in.

For more information on hydrating foods, EZ water, and Quench:

https://bit.ly/Quech101

9

Nitric Oxide: 'Talk Right'

"A cell with unfettered access to information never becomes diseased" – Zach Bush MD

Poor communication is a major cause of stress. Between nations, between people, and even inside of you, such as between the brain and your organs.

Communication can be split into external communication (i.e. outwards to other people) and internal communication. External communication is an extension of 'Think Right' as are aspects of internal communication (how we 'talk' to ourselves).

There are entire books written on these communication subjects, and some great online courses (I have two 'Think Right' courses available online as it's such a huge subject), so for this book I'll focus on one very important internal aspect of communication.

Optimal internal communication is critical to health. Unfortunately, many of today's lifestyle choices and pressures disrupt our internal communication systems. Even most medicine (even something as 'harmless' as Calpol – which is also known as paracetamol or Tylenol) can have a disastrous effect on communication.

As well as your internal thoughts, other aspects of internal communication include:

- your nerves (which is why chiropractic can help some people with high blood pressure)
- your hormones
- your brain chemicals known as neurotransmitters
- your endocannabinoid system (yes, cannabis system)
- light (we actually make light and use it to communicate inside us)
- many other 'chemical messenger systems'

It is one of these chemical messenger systems that is particularly significant for those with high blood pressure.

It's a chemical called nitric oxide.

Nitric oxide:

- Protects your heart by relaxing your blood vessels and normalising your blood pressure
- Stimulates your brain, which can impact behaviour
- Kills bacteria
- Defends against tumour cells
- Helps combat diabetes
- Aids in oxygen delivery and therefore energy production (great for athletes)

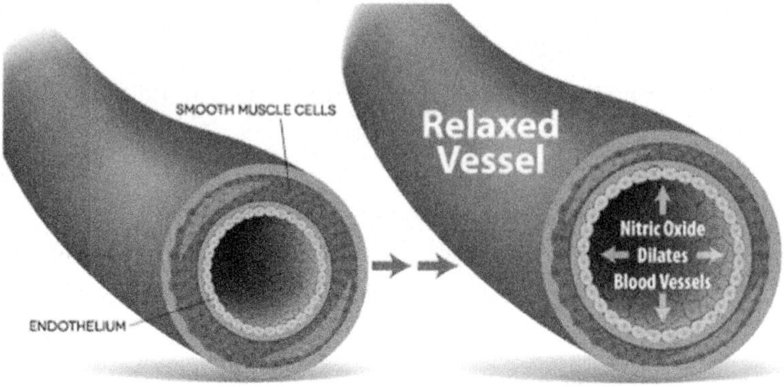

Nitric oxide, quite simply abbreviated to NO, is a magic molecule we all make that helps dilate blood vessels, aids our health in numerous ways, and helps in keeping us happy!

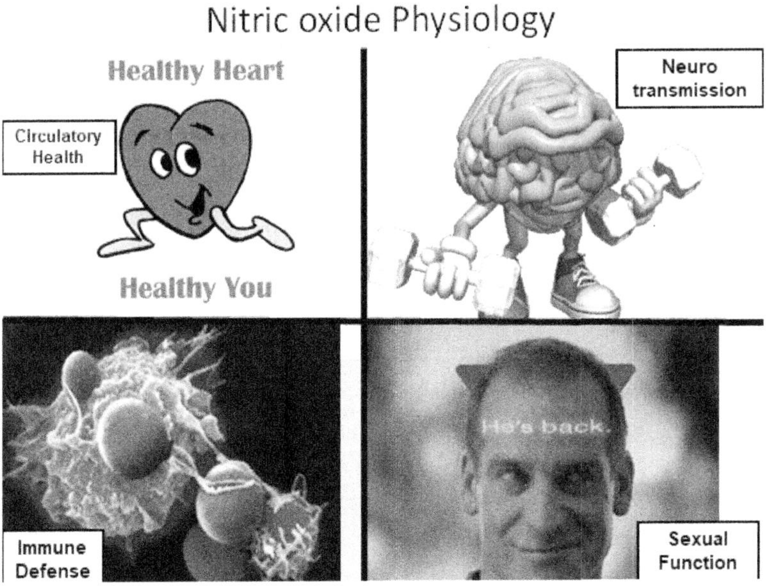

There are a number of strategies you can use to improve and optimise nitric oxide levels in your body including supplements, food, breathing techniques and certain exercises.

You do not however want to boost it without control, which is why one of my favourite strategies is to use a specific medicinal mushroom called Ganoderma Lucidum – and a very specific brand as well.

As I think nitric oxide control is so important I have prepared a great resource you can download here, which includes foods, recipes, supplements, a link to the specific ones I use, and more, all for free: www.nitric.gr8.com

Here are the basics though...

There are 2 main supplements promoted to help raise nitric oxide: arginine and l-citruline. It's also recommended to get lots of natural nitrates from food.

I recommend stating with a 'Nitric Oxide' intense diet for 7 days before trying supplements (as there are many other benefits from having a healthy eating plan).

For arginine:

Turkey, Pork, chicken, fish, sesame seeds, pumpkin seeds, spinach , watercress, eggs, soybeans, walnuts, chickpeas, lentils
i.e.For most meat eaters it is unlikely you are arginine deficient.

For L-citrulline:

Watermelon really does stand out as the only true way to boost citrulline without supplements.

These will all help: cucumber is easy to eat in high quantities , onions, liver, salmon, almonds, walnuts, pomegranate, rocket (arugula)

For Nitrates:

Rocket, spinach, lettuce, beetroot, radish -4x 80g servings a day

For Nitric Oxide Protection and Increased Production:

Pomegranate, black ginger root (if you can find it) and the medicinal mushroom ganoderma lucidum (see above). Garlic will also help NO production.

All citrus fruits help protect the NO you have. So good old oranges! (the whole orange, not the juice by itself)

For Nitric Oxide Control:

Chia seeds, moringa powder, raspberries, cherries.

Bonus: Dark chocolate (see below for amount)

Other Foods That May Help

Brown rice has been shown to significantly lower inflammatory markers associated with heart disease. I would certainly suggest swapping white rice and pasta to brown rice to help lose weight, and improve your health in general.

Cranberries, Cranberry juice and Cranberry powder have shown heart health benefits, including nitric oxide production that lowered blood pressure (in rats anyway!)

Honey has been shown to improve nitric oxide production in rats. Personally I love honey, and used to keep my own bees, so I really hope it's going to be proved in humans too.

<u>Specific minimum amounts needed to make a real difference in your body</u>

Drinking 100ml of beetroot juice will increase NO in your blood in 45 min.

Eating 400g of spinach, rocket or watercress (or other high nitrate plants) every day for 1 week will increase oxygen flow by 20%. Salivary NO increase 8x after just one meal.

30g of dark chocolate for 15 days!

Quick Fix

Simply try adding 1 nitric oxide smoothie/juice and 1 nitric oxide salad to your diet every day.

For Meat Eaters

If you are a meat eater it is unlikely you are lacking arginine, but I would urge you to try cutting out all meat for 7 days, and sticking to fish and plant based sources of arginine, and let me know how you feel.

While arginine is a mainstay of nitric oxide supplements you will probably get more benefits from concentrating on increasing nitrate rich foods especially if you are a meat eater.

For Vegetarians and Vegans

For vegetarians, try a week of really focusing on raising arginine and citrulline, while also making sure that your veggie diet really is rich in nitrates too.

Smoothies

A quick note on flavour – I often use a flavoured fruit and vegetable powder from Nutri-Dyn - available in North America and the UK.

Smoothies are a great way to get what you need in a convenient way for breakfast, lunch or dinner.

As a very basic way to ensure you have adequate nitrates and NO boosters, find a good source or organic freshly squeezed beetroot and pomegranate juice and drink a 100ml glass of each every day.

Nitrate and Arginine

- 200 ml pomegranate or cherry juice
- 1 frozen banana (peel and chop before freezing – or keep the peel on if it's organic)
- 4 tbs sesame seeds (for the arginine)
- 1 beetroot (peeled and roughly chopped)
- 100g of spinach
- 100 g Mixed berries (I like to use frozen)
- Water as needed

Nitrate and Citrulline

- 1 cup of beetroot juice
- ¼ to ½ watermelon
- 1 cup pomegranate juice
- 1-inch piece of ginger, peeled and sliced
- Water as needed

Citrulline

- 4 cups seedless watermelon (diced)
- 4 cups frozen strawberries
- 2 tablespoons lime juice
- 6 fresh mint leaves (large)

Citrulline and NO protection

- 2 cups watermelon (cubed)
- 1 cup fresh raspberries
- 1 cup frozen blueberries
- 1 cup ice

For more resources: www.nitric.gr8.com

10

Modified Mediterranean 'Paleo NO' DASH Diet: Eat Right

"Let food be thy medicine and medicine be thy food."
Hippocrates, the founder of modern medicine

"The food you eat can be either the safest and most powerful form of medicine or the slowest form of poison" Ann Wigmore

So, are you eating yourself to death or are you eating yourself to life?

The choice is yours, but you may not have been taught what the best choices may be.

The number one key is ensuring you have a variety of different plant-based foods in your diet, and the magic number is 30. This if from the Predict Study on twins. Having at least 30 different plants in your diet every week was hugely beneficial to health.

The better the diversity of plants, the better, healthier and more diverse are the friendly bacteria that live inside you (probiotics). And the Predict Study found that gut bacteria health (microbiome health) was MORE important than genetics when it came to the health of identical twins.

So that's vegetables, fruits, berries, nuts, seeds, spices and herbs.

Another big factor tied directly to plant food intake is fibre.

Even if you already eat a lot of fibre, your health could be improved by eating more!

If you find it initially difficult to get enough plant variety and fibre there are some fantastic 'fruit and vegetable' powdered drinks and fibre powders available.

For some, this makes transitioning much easier (and I use one specific brand of delicious flavoured greens drink myself as I like it so much)

<u>Best Specific Healthy Eating Plan</u>

There are a number of diets proven to help improve blood pressure, the one with the most science to back it up is the up to date DASH diet with its Mediterranean update.

DASH is short for Dietary Approaches to Stop Hypertension.

You can make the DASH diet more 'Paleo', and certainly look at incorporating foods from the Nitric Oxide Diet.

There are other options which when I work with clients we can find the right one.

<u>A Possible Problem With a 'Good Food Alone' Approach</u>

Drugs can have dramatic effects as they are thousands of times more powerful than many natural substances they are based on (which is why they can be like adding a hurricane to your body, when you may only needed a gentle breeze). As people often want fast results, food and lifestyle alone may not be fast enough to bring about changes and this is where supplements can help.

There are two books that really helped me become certain of this need to supplement in the modern age, especially if you are suffering with a chronic health condition.

The first is Health Defence by Dr. Paul Clayton.

In it he references a study that looked at the health span and lifespan of people in Victorian England:

"Analysis of the mid-Victorian period in the U.K. reveals that life expectancy at age 5 was as good or better than exists today, and the incidence of degenerative disease was 10% of ours... they consumed levels of micro- and phytonutrients at approximately ten times the levels considered normal today." Form Int. J. Environ. Res. Public Health. 2009 Mar;6(3):1235-53. PMID: 19440443

Did you get that? The Victorian diet had ten times the nutrients (not calories) we have today.

So why do we live longer now than in Victorian times?

Well in Health Defence Dr.Clayton looks deeper at this, and found that it really came down to surviving the first 4 years of life. If someone in Victorian England made it for 4 years old, they where likely to then be healthy into their seventies, and have a lifespan close to ours.

A 'health span' into the seventies is far better than our current health span.

The second book is the intriguingly titled "Healing Is Voltage: The Handbook." By Dr Jerry Tennant.

Here's an extract:

"*the body is constantly wearing itself out and having to make new cells. You get new cones in the macula of your eye every 48 hours. The lining of the gut is replaced every three days. The skin that you and I are sitting in today is only 6 weeks old. Your liver's 8 weeks old. Your nervous system's 8 months old.*

One of the things I began to realize then is that chronic disease only occurs when you lose the ability to make new cells that work"

In the book Dr Tennant speak about the need for 'sick cells' of nutrients and 'voltage' is many times greater than the need of healthy cells.

I explain it to my patients with a house analogy.

To keep a home in good condition it may need the occasion light bulb change, a new layer of paint every few years, a few roof tiles replaced. Basically, not much time, energy or raw materials.

However, if your house suffers major storm damage, or if you let it decay, then a wall may collapse, or the roof cave in. This may require scaffolding, and a lot more time, work and expense.

In the same way, if you are 'sick' you may require many times more nutrients than someone who is healthy. Although keep in mind, looking at the Victorian study, we may need many times more nutrients to stay optimally healthy than we currently think.

There are other studies looking at the benefits of nutrition over food, one more is simply titled '*Food is too weak*'. As Dr Bob Rakowski puts it "Food is too weak to replete depleted cells & bodies".

Here's part of the report:

"improvement in nutritional behavior could not replenish already exhausted nutrient reservoirs. Only supplementation was able to significantly boost nutrient levels and confer beneficial effects on general welfare, physical performance, and resistance to infections. Therefore, it appears that nutritional supplements are advisable for everyone", you can find it here: Advances in Therapy, Volume 24, Number 5 / September, 2007

<u>A mineral for optimal blood pressure</u>

"Magnesium deficiency intensifies adverse reactions to stress that can be life threatening. Such reactions are mediated by excess release of the stress hormones: catecholamines and corticosteroids - which are increased by low Mg" Int Journal of the American College of Nutrition, Vol. 13, No. 5, 429-446 (1994)

Magnesium deficiency is very prevalent and can lead to high blood pressure, it can also lead to lots of muscle tension and cramps, it is also related to low immunity boor blood sugar control and poor bowel function.

So along with a good diet, and a multivitamin, extra magnesium supplementation is a great place to start for people with high blood pressure.

It's hard to overdose on magnesium because your bowels will get rid of it. Start off with a small dose and slowly increase it to your bowel tolerance, then back off a bit, very simple. (By bowel tolerance I mean until your bowels start rumbling or you get loose stools).

There are a number of different forms of magnesium available.

For instance, Magnesium Oxide is the most poorly absorbed, so most likely to cause bowel issues. Magnesium threonate is possibly the best absorbed, and best for the brain.

Magnesium taurate is also very good for the brain. Magnesium malate is often used for muscle soreness. And magnesium citrate and glycinate are also good options for blood pressure.

I personally vary which type I take (except I never use the oxide version!)

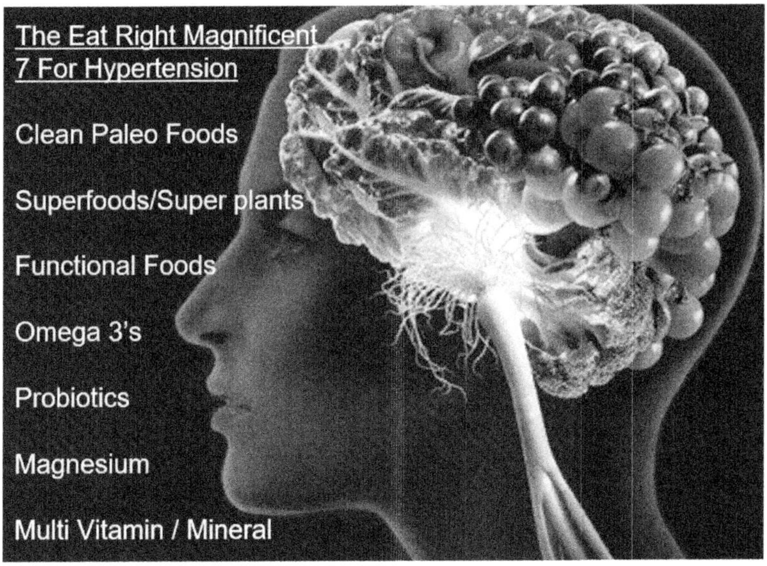
The Eat Right Magnificent
7 For Hypertension
Clean Paleo Foods
Superfoods/Super plants
Functional Foods
Omega 3's
Probiotics
Magnesium
Multi Vitamin / Mineral

11

Detox 'the 10 Day Blood Pressure Blitz'

Imagine your current state of health is like a car stuck in the mud.

You can spin the wheels as fast as you want and nothing happens (ie you are leading a healthy lifestyle but you don't feel well - or you feel fine but have high blood pressure)

You ask a friend to give you a push, but that's not enough (you add in supplements that others have told you worked for them).

You get a large group of people to push you or a tow truck to pull you out, and that does the job (the power of true detox!).

'Poop Right' in the Magnificent 7 is not just about the bowels – it's about all of our detoxification processes. So it includes liver health, kidney health, the health of our individual cells, and even our skin (are you sweating enough?).

Environmental toxins are one of the biggest, and most under treated, causes of high blood pressure. Everything from the polluted air we breathe, to pesticides and herbicides in our food have been proven to be causative factors in blood pressure problems, and unless you take steps to avoid and remove them no amount of other healthy lifestyle habits will help.

You may think you have a clean environment because you live in the countryside, but did you know that even for the Inuit Indians living in Northern Canada, one of the cleanest, most remote environments on the planet, there is a link between Persistent Organic Pollutants 'POPS' and high blood pressure?

Even whales living in the Pacific Ocean are exposed to air pollution!

If you live much nearer civilisation, and especially if you live in a big town or city, or near a factory or power plant, you will 100% be at risk from air pollution.

Has your doctor taken this into consideration and given you the necessary steps to clean up your body, and clean the air around you?

There are multiple avenues for toxins to get into your body, from inheriting lead pollution from your mother, to various other heavy metals through second hand smoke, pesticides, herbicides, chemicals from new mattresses, and mould exposure from an old leak, or poorly looked after bathroom.

Toxins are a very real cause of multiple health issues, yet for some reason medical doctors are not being taught how to identify or deal will this far reaching set of problems.

As well as doing things to decrease your toxic exposure, such as buying a quality air filter, and filling your home with plants, there are multiple detox pathways you can optimise in your body.

One of the processes I recommend to all my patients is the '7 Day Reboot', a very effective detoxification protocol I learned from Dr Bob Rakowski.

We have also developed a '10 Day Blood Pressure Blitz' and use a longer 90 day detox program to clean deep into the brain.

Detoxification is a process that is going on all the time in our bodies so needs constant attention.

As deep detoxification can be a challenge, and is best done with guidance I've developed a 5 day training course using some basic, safe approaches.

If you have access to the internet please feel free to join: https://bit.ly/detox5lb

The reason I have not published the '10 Day Blood Pressure Blitz' is that it does vary a little from patient to patient AND I don't want to accidentally suggest something extreme that may interfere with your medication for other health issues.

12

Resilience to Stress: Think Right

"The greatest discovery of any generation is that human beings can alter their lives by altering the attitude of their minds."
Albert Schweitzer (Nobel Peace Prize Winner)

"Your health today is the result of the decisions you made in the past. Your health tomorrow is the result of the decisions you make today."
Me, based on a quote from Buddha

"The brain can be developed just the same as the muscles can be developed... it can be strengthened by proper exercise and proper use. By developing your thinking powers you expand the capacity of your brain and attain new abilities."
Thomas Edison

"You will never change your life until you change something you do daily. The secret of your success is found in your daily routine."
John C. Maxwell

"Do something you hate everyday, just for the practice."
John C. Maxwell

Right now, you have the chance to make some very different decisions about the future of your health because you can learn to 'think right' and make different decisions.

If you think that changing your thinking is difficult here's a quote from one of my heroes that explains my approach:

"If you want to teach people a new way of thinking, don't bother trying to teach them instead, give them a tool, the use of which will lead to new ways of thinking."
Richard Buckminster Fuller

And so when I teach the Magnificent 7 health strategies, 'Thinking Tools' are often the place I start.

In my training courses, I teach four types of thinking tool,

1. tools to help understand yourself
2. tools to help change yourself
3. tools to make you more resilient (to stress)
4. tools that move you forward

Some Thinking Tools

6 Phase Meditation (Vishen Lakhiani)

Psychocybernetics (Maxwell Maltz

Mi365 – Pete Cohen

Affirmations - Marissa Peer 'I am enough'

Breathing techniques

QUESTIONS

Self Knowing/Self Analysis

Food

Supplements

Movement/Exercise

Detox

Alpha Music (John Levine)

Socialising

'Brain Tap' & Heart Math technology

When it comes to blood pressure, probably the most important tools are the ones that help you build resilience to stress and decrease anxiety.

Bullet proofing yourself to stress is the science of hormesis.

Hormesis is a word I heard of first from Ari Whitten, author of Eat For Energy, and developer of the Energy Blueprint online course.

The Stress-Brain Loop

Chronic stress, even from seemingly normal events like watching the news and suffering repeated tiny bouts of emotional stress, mixed with bad days at work, and inadequate sleep set of changes in our brain and hormones that lead to decreased:

- attention
- perception
- short-term memory
- learning ability

Which all adds up to more stress and increased:

- blood sugar
- blood pressure

So one of the first tools I teach chronically stressed people is something called 'The Physiological Sigh'.

I first learned this super-simple breathing technique from Ari Whitten.

The Physiological Sigh breaks the stress loop.

All you have to do is take a deep breath in through the nose, and then a second short, quick extra breath in like a sniff to pump up your lungs even more. You then breath slowly out, and can even make a sighing sound.

Just doing this once can be enough, but 2 or 3 times in a row is better.

You may have noticed people breathe a little like this naturally when they are crying. In fact all mammals have this built in pattern of breathing that kicks in at certain times, including while we sleep.

If my explanation above is not clear enough, it's easy to find on Youtube. I've done one myself, after I combined the Physiological Sigh with 2 other techniques and renamed it 'Zen breathing' because of the particularly powerful effect is has on chilling out the mind.

You can learn here: https://bit.ly/zenbreath

While many of the thinking tools are active (ie you have to do something) there are some passive ones to. The one we use in the clinic is Alpha Music, developed by John Levine.

Alpha Music has been used in hospitals and has been shown to speed up healing. It soothes the brain directly and all you have to do is play it in the background, or on headphones.

You can pick up some Alpha Music on John's website:
www.tinyurl.com/amofjohn

There are plenty more tools to build resilience and bust stress and very often it's all about finding the ones you like doing. Check out the resources section at the end of the book.

More here - https://bit.ly/mag7brain

13

Circadian Rhythm: Better Sleep

"AMAZING BREAKTHROUGH!

Scientists have discovered a revolutionary new treatment that makes you live longer. It enhances your memory and makes you more creative. It makes you look more attractive. It keeps you slim and lowers food cravings. It protects you from cancer and dementia. It wards off colds and the flu. It lowers your risk of heart attacks and strokes, not to mention diabetes. You'll even feel happier, less depressed, and less anxious. Are you interested?"

"The physical and mental impairments caused by one night of bad sleep dwarf those caused by an equivalent absence of food or exercise."

Matthew Walker PhD, in 'Why We Sleep'

Did you know 40% of women and 25% of men have sleep problems?

DID YOU KNOW HEART ATTACKS AND TRAFFIC ACCIDENTS SPIKE THE DAY AFTER WE THE CLOCKS GO FORWARD EVERY YEAR?

Your brain cleans up cellular garbage when you sleep.

Your body repairs itself while you sleep.

It's important!

I'll explain the term circadian rhythm shortly. First, let's talk about sleep.

Sleep is not merely a "time out" from our busy routines; it is essential for quality of life.

Sleep is something our "mind-body" needs for resetting, restoring, refreshing and replenishing.

When you sleep, your brain cleans up its cellular garbage and your body repairs itself.

You can be eating and exercising perfectly, and you can be supplementing with nutrients, but if you're not sleeping enough, your body isn't going to repair. If your arteries are damaged (which happens on a daily basis) and you don't get enough sleep this can lead to high blood pressure.

What Does Sleep Do For You?

- Improves the function of the nervous system
- Prevents or reverses depression
- Restores hormone imbalances
- Increases concentration
- Boosts the immune system
- Significantly reduces cholesterol
- Improves learning a memory
- Maintains emotional harmony

So sleep is free, it just takes time, and it's very important. If you are having sleep problems, then you have a major health problem, and I'd urge you to work on this right away.

There are a number of strategies I use with my patients to improve sleep, and sometimes it needs some serious coaching.

Here are a few simple tips:

- A good mattress
- The right pillow
- A quiet, dark, cool room to sleep in
- Relax for at least one hour before going to bed.
- Optimise nitric oxide
- Adequate magnesium intake
- Get the right light at the right time of day - see below...

The title of this chapter is 'circadian rhythm' so what does that mean?

Circadian rhythms are regularly recurring, biological changes in our mental and physical behaviours over the course of the day and are primarily controlled by our body's innate intelligence, our biological "clock."

Research shows that these rhythms occur in processes such as blood pressure, body temperature, hormone levels, and the immune system.

Circadian rhythms are the natural rhythms that wake us up in the morning and help us sleep at night.

And the best way to help so many people in today's 'artificial light' society is to reintroduce them to sunshine.

Did you know that sunshine helps convert cholesterol to vitamin D3? And that sunshine helps lower blood pressure? And one of the keys to getting better sleep is getting some early morning sun?

I first really learned about circadian rhythms from Ari Whitten (again!)

The specific aspect of light to focus on is blue light.

Morning daylight is full of blue light, which we only really benefit from if we are outside (even sitting in a bright room next to a window on a sunny day is not as good as getting outside on a cloudy day).

Blue light is what triggers our pineal gland 'timer' inside our brain to lower melatonin in the day, and then later in the day to raise melatonin.

Melatonin is known as the 'sleep hormone' (it does much more than this though).

When mid-day comes, the sun is overhead and this also tells us it's daytime and to stay awake.

The trouble is, most of the screens we now watch are pumping out more blue light – smart phones, computer screens and TV screens.

Also many of today's light bulbs and LED lights are geared to blue light – so if we get home in the evening and turn on overhead lighting our brain is tricked into thinking its mid-day again!

All this artificial blue light and overhead light exposure severely depletes night time melatonin production which means poor quality sleep, and poor repair and recovery.

A simple 'hack' is to spend at least 10 minutes outside as early as possible in the day, get out side again for a few minutes at mid-day, and then to turn off all overhead lights in the evening, and to invest in some blue light blocking glasses to wear in the evening too. (You'll find lots online).

Alternatively – get up at dawn, and get to bed by 8pm!

14

The Goldilocks Exercise Program

"Physical inactivity produces an abnormal gene expression and is a direct causal factor of most chronic health conditions"
F.W.Booth Ph.D.

3 Important Facts About Exercise:

1. Exercise normalises gene expression. Normal gene expression = health.
2. Movement stimulates the brain, which in turn looks after our vital organs, muscles and psychological well-being.
3. It raises a very important chemical in our bodies known as glutathione.
   Glutathione is an antioxidant which in basic terms means it prevents us from rusting from the inside. (see below)

According to the Mayo Clinic in the USA, regular physical activity — such as 150 minutes a week, or about 30 minutes most days of the week — can lower your blood pressure by about 5 to 8 mm Hg if you have high blood pressure.

The quickest way to get across how important exercise is, is to understand how important a glutathione is.

Glutathione is something we all make in our bodies, and it's boosted by having the right nutrients AND the right amount of exercise.

And the easiest way to realise the importance of glutathione is to have a look at this this graphic:

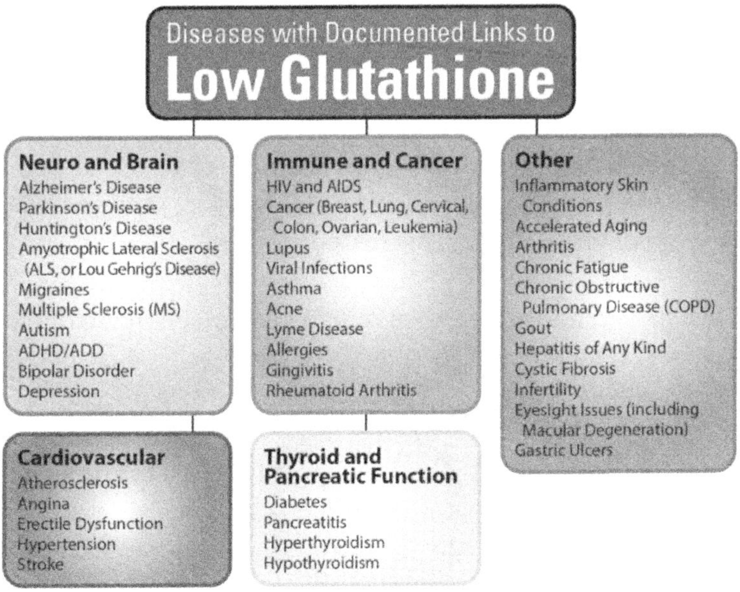

Diseases with Documented Links to
Low Glutathione
Neuro and Brain
Alzheimer's Disease
Parkinson's Disease
Huntington's Disease
Amyotrophic Lateral Sclerosis (ALS, or Lou Gehrig's Disease)
Migraines
Multiple Sclerosis (MS)
Autism
ADHD/ADD
Bipolar Disorder
Depression
Immune and Cancer
HIV and AIDS
Cancer (Breast, Lung, Cervical, Colon, Ovarian, Leukemia)
Lupus
Viral Infections
Asthma
Acne
Lyme Disease
Allergies
Gingivitis
Rheumatoid Arthritis
Other
Inflammatory Skin Conditions
Accelerated Aging
Arthritis
Chronic Fatigue
Chronic Obstructive Pulmonary Disease (COPD)
Gout
Hepatitis of Any Kind
Cystic Fibrosis
Infertility
Eyesight Issues (including Macular Degeneration)
Gastric Ulcers
Cardiovascular
Atherosclerosis
Angina
Erectile Dysfunction
Hypertension
Stroke
Thyroid and Pancreatic Function
Diabetes
Pancreatitis
Hyperthyroidism
Hypothyroidism

(I found this image on the internet many years ago – if you know the owner please let me know so I can credit them)

If you exercise too much though, you can deplete glutathione, which can be disastrous, not just because of the above, but because it's very important in conjunction with nitric oxide.

One of the biggest mistakes 'very fit' people make is exercising beyond their capacity to recycle glutathione – which is why 'ultra-fit' endurance athletes can suddenly develop autoimmune bowel conditions, or have a heart attack after a marathon despite no previous signs of heart disease, or develop serious Covid 19 issues.

It's not just glutathione that is depleted by overexercise, it's your entire ability to recover, repair, burn fat at rest, and grow muscle.

This is why I put exercise last on the list here, and why I guide my patients and clients to the 'just right' amount of exercise for them. Just like Goldilocks.

If you suffer with high blood pressure and you exercise lots, then maybe try easing up, try something less damaging to your body like yoga or Pilates instead of cross-fit 4 x week.

If you have don't exercise then find more OTM's – 'opportunities to move' through the day and try something gradual like the Couch to 5k program.

If the reason you can't exercise is because of pain, then find a physiotherapist, osteopath or chiropractor who specialises in getting people moving again – there is almost always some way to get more movement in your life.

More on our website about glutathione: https://bit.ly/glutathione-health

I'll end this chapter with a quote from Dr James Chestnut:

"If you are deficient in exercise you are unable to utilize food nutrients properly. If you are nutritionally deficient you are unable to utilize exercise properly."

15

Health Span vs Life Span

A final thought for you.

So at the beginning, I mentioned adding 20 years of health to your life.

You may have heard of the life span, which is the average age we live to, which in the UK is about 82.

But what's your health span?

Here's a slide from one of Dr Rakowski's presentations:

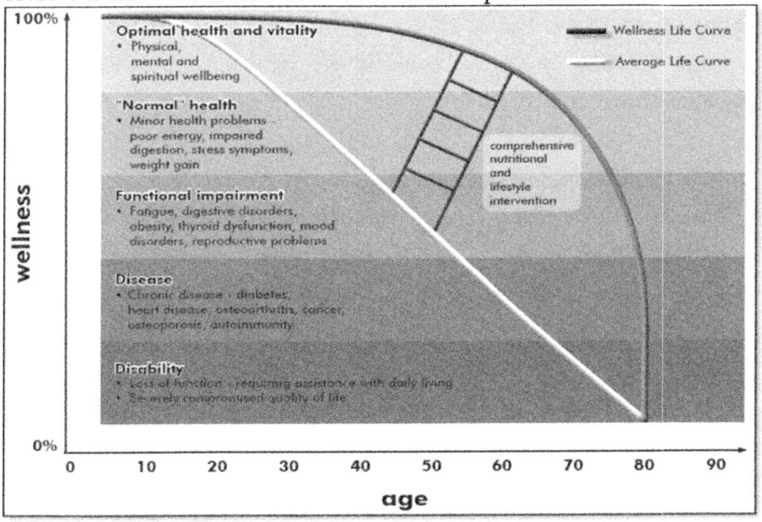

Your health span is how long you will be alive before you're on drugs for the rest of your life; due to a chronic, most likely preventable, health problem.

It may surprise you to know that even though life span has increased over the past 40 years, our average health span is about the same as it was 40, 50, 60 years ago. Even more surprising, our modern health span is actually worse than it was about a 120 years ago in Victorian England (as long as you made it to the age of 4 that is).

The average health span today in the UK is between 50 and 60 depending on where you live. Which is that same as in the 1950's.

So most people can expect to enjoy at least 25 years of declining health and disability with symptoms being suppressed by drugs, but not much actual improvement.

However, there are those, that may not live much longer than the average lifespan of 82, but they have a health span of 80. That's 20 years more quality life!

The good news is that although it may take 30 years to produce trillions of sick cells – enough to cause an illness or symptom like high blood pressure, and it takes years to replace them all with cells that replicate healthy cells, you can start your journey back to a longer health span fairly swiftly, and at any time.

All you have to do is start implementing the Magnificent 7 health strategies.

When implemented correctly the 'Magnificent 7' process you can expect to:

- Reduce body fat, tone up and get leaner

- Have more energy and feel better about yourself
- Develop a bulletproof mindset
- Have freedom with your nutrition, break free from calorie counting and worrying what to eat and not eat
- Become fitter and stronger and reduce risk of high blood pressure, heart disease, diabetes and many other preventable illnesses

III

The Assessment & Resources

16

The Magnificent 7 Lifestyle Screening Assessment

You can download a copy here: https://bit.ly/mag7screen

Please read carefully as how you answer the 'Think Right' and 'Move Right' questions is in reverse to the other 5 sections.

For the Think and Move sections (Part 1 and 2) tick 0 for strongly agree, and 2 for strongly disagree, and 1 for somewhere in between

For the rest it is 2 for strongly agree, and 0 for strongly disagree, and 1 for somewhere in between

So – the lower your score the better! Be honest with yourself...

Think Right

	0 (Agree)	1	2
Life is rewarding, I am optimistic about the future			
I find beauty and joy in things and laugh often			
It is more important that I enjoy what I do, rather than if people are impressed by it			
I get intensely involved in, and feel greatly fulfilled by, many of the things I do each day			
I never get stressed or overwhelmed			

Total Score _____

Move Right

	0 (Agree)	1	2
I walk 45 minutes every day			
I move all my joints every day, in every direction			
I lift weights/strength train 2 x week or more			
I regularly stretch			
I get out of breath and sweat from exercise 2x week or more			

Total Score _____

REMEMBER: For the rest it is 2 for strongly agree, and 0 for strongly disagree, and 1 for somewhere in between

Inner Communication (Talk Right)

	0	1	2 (Agree)
I have a thyroid problem			
I think I have hormone balance problem (male or female)			
I suffer with fatigue			
Feeling of depression or sadness			
I have 'problems with my nerves' (either pain related, or anxiety)			
Regular Muscle cramps			
Heart arrhythmias			

Total Score _____

Eat Right

	0	1	2 (Agree)
Crave sweets and/or carbohydrates			
Irritable/headaches/fatigue or other symptoms between meals			
Poor nails, skin or hair			
Bleeding gums or easily bruised			
Muscle cramps			
Bloating or heartburn/acid reflux			

Total Score _____

Hydrate Right

	0	1	2 (Agree)
I DON'T drink water between meals			
Frequently thirsty			
Dry skin/eyes/lips/mouth or throat			
I DON'T exercise regularly			

Total Score _____

Sleep Right

	0	1	2 (Agree)
Less than 6 hours of sleep a night			
Disturbed sleep			
Hard to get to sleep			
Hard to wake up			
Fall asleep in under 10 min even during the day			

Total Score _____

Detox Right

	0	1	2 (Agree)
Constipation or diarrhea			
I take regular medication			
General itchiness			
Sensitive to strong smells			
Live near heavy traffic/industrial plant/live in a city			
Exposure to chemicals (including cleaning chemicals)			
Chronic aches/pains/skin problems			

Total Score _____

GRAND TOTAL _________

<u>Results Interpretation</u>

<u>Single Questions:</u>

If you scored yourself a 2 on any one single question then I'd urge you to investigate further - as it may be the beginning of something that at the moment is preventable. If you leave it to long though it may develop into a chronic condition and interfere with your quality of life.

This is especially important in the Sleep section.

If you are already taking medication 'for the rest of your life', regardless of the rest of your scores, your systems have already 'broken', most likely (but not always) from lifestyle. We work with many people who have been put on drugs 'for life' and when they make the right changes they can actually heal and get off them.

Single Section:

If you scored 4 or more in any one of the 7 sections then you will almost certainly benefit from improving lifestyle habits in that area.

If you scored 6 or more in any one section you will benefit by making changes today! You may want to reach out to a health coach or give your doctor a call.

Total Score:

0-21: Pretty good, and you will know where you need to improve and optimize.

22- 35: Start making some lifestyle changes. Maybe do some deeper investigation with someone involved in natural/functional/integrative health.

36 or above: Lifestyle is a major issue, you probably already know that, and it's time to seek some help, take action, implement changes, and take self-health responsibility.

Acknowledgments

This assessment is mostly a simplified version of Dr Bryan Walsh's Cell Blueprint TM which consists of 30 sections – and I use with my 1 to 1 and coaching clients as part of a more in-depth assessment.

The ‘Magnificent 7 Health Strategies’ is an original concept from Dr Bob Rakowski

17

What's Next?

Well if you have not already taken some action, take the Magnificent 7 Lifestyle Assessment, and start where indicated.

As I mentioned at the start, you can reach out to me or take advantage of some of the free resources online.

The 5 Day, 5lb Detox: https://bit.ly/detox5lb

Zen Breathing: https://bit.ly/zenbreath

Hydrate Right: https://bit.ly/Quech101

Nitric Oxide Resources: www.nitric.gr8.com

Alpha Music: www.tinyurl.com/amofjohn

Brain Based Wellness: https://bit.ly/mag7brain

Glutathione and Health; https://bit.ly/glutathione-health

Magnificent 7 Health Screen Download: https://bit.ly/mag7screen

My hope is that you found this book useful, and the advice was clear enough to take action on.

If you found it useful it would help me, and help others if you left a favourable review on Amazon.

Thank you for reading and I wish you the best of health.

18

About the Author

Chris Pickard D.C, B.Sc, a functional health consultant, started learning about health and wellness from Dr. Deepak Chopra at 17 when he learned to meditate. He went on to become a chiropractor and became fascinated with the relationship between the mind, the nervous system and immunity.

After graduating he realized the need to learn more about nutrition to help his patients even more.

This eventually lead him to learn from some of the world's top functional nutrition and detox practitioners in the USA, including Dr Bob Rakowski, Dr Dan Pompa, Dr Bryan Walsh, and the renowned cardiologist Dr Jack Wolfson to become the first trained Holistic Heart Health practitioner in the UK.

As well as working with Olympic Gold Medalists, martial arts World Champions, and those who have lost hope, he is also the expert many health practitioners go to when they need help with their own nutrition, mindset and well being.

Printed in Great Britain
by Amazon

37279075R00050